Contents

1. Introduction — 1

2. History Of Garlic - Why It Works — 4

3. The Power Of Garlic — 12

4. Anti-aging Superfood — 15

5. Cautions — 21

6. Conclusion — 22

Disclaimer — 23

GARLIC - ANTI-AGING MEDICINE YOU MAY BUY IN THE SUPERMARKET

ONE OF THE MOST POWERFUL SUPERFOODS SINCE THE AGE OF THE PHARAOHS REDISCOVERED

MARCUS D. ADAMS

ISBN 978-1-63940-289-2

ONE

INTRODUCTION

At the age of 40, our bodies start aging at a faster rate than they had to that point. Studies have shown that without the proper nutrients and exercise, our bodies are aging about 6 months extra for every year that passes! So, let's say you're 40. By the time you reach 50, you will look and feel 55. By the time you reach 60, you will look and feel 70 years old! I don't know about you but that kind of aging does not appeal to me a whole lot.

Did you ever notice that the folks who stay the most physically active seem to be aging more slowly than others who don't? In my mind, I picture a 63-year old woman gardening while her 65-year-old husband is chopping wood nearby and they both look like they're in their 50s. Hmm... maybe that was a scene from a 1940s movie but I think it makes the point. They kept active with muscle taxing activities and no doubt felt and looked younger because of it. Steve Holman says that 90% of people over the age of 35 lose enough muscle every year to burn off an additional 4 pounds of body fat. The aging process really starts to catch up with us at that point. Muscle gives shape and strength to our bodies. As we know, when you lose muscle mass, you gain fat, even if the calories you take in stay the same. We don't feel or look as good. Then we get depressed because we don't feel and look as good. Then we give up on retaining our youth and it's all downhill from there. Wow. That was depressing, huh?

As you age, different processes in your skin change its appearance, activity and structure. The aging skin has reduced cellular activity, less collagen production, lowered epidermal turn over and damage accumulation as a result of free radicals from UV exposure. All these changes contribute to the aging process and leave you with apparent signs of aging such as wrinkles, fine lines and dark spots. They come about because the skin loses moisture and elasticity from all the aging changes

Causes of premature skin aging

What most people don't know is that the aging process can actually be slowed by living healthy lifestyles. This way, you won't have to start using anti-aging products until much later in life. When you take good care of the skin, you will prevent premature aging, which results from things such as;

- Psychological stress
- Unhealthy diets
- Nicotine
- Excessive alcohol consumption
- UV radiation

All these factors put you at risk of free radical formation leading to premature skin aging. A few lifestyle changes might be all you need to maintain a youthful look before it is time to use a wrinkle cream. To block out sun damage, you can use a day cream and sunscreen.

Fear not! That doesn't have to happen.

This accelerated aging is reversible because, there are specific ways to move and eat that will slow down the rapid aging process to the point where you're aging less than a year for every year. That means we can look younger in a few years than we do now? Now that is an aging plan we could get behind, right?

HISTORY OF GARLIC - WHY IT WORKS

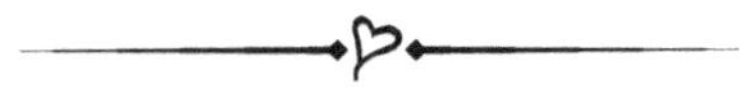

Garlic has been used by people for centuries. From Mesopotamia to ancient Egypt to Babylon, the Greeks to Medieval times and up through our modern era its benefits have been observed and scientifically proven. Medical history records the medicinal effects of garlic have been consistent and in use as medicine as a diuretic, digestive aid, antibiotic, antiparacitic, anti-congestant, to soothe continuous coughing, clearing arteries, treat asthma, colds, edema, and cancer prevention among other uses for ?uite some time.

Because of garlic's recognized importance as a fantastic aid to health in history and its newly discovered significance for our generation, garlic's chemistry has been well researched. Literally hundreds of compounds interact within garlic to make it one of the best health foods of history and modern times. The sulfur compounds work to interfere with many bad compounds that cause viral and bacterial infections, cancers, cholesterol, blood clots etc.

References to garlic can be found throughout history but in 1562 the first valid work on herbs by William Turner, herbalist to Queen Elizabeth I, was published as William Turner's New Herbal. In 1812 garlic was used extensively by doctors in England and can be found in Jonathan Stoke's, A Botanical Material Medical. It lists comments on garlic from over forty medical books of the time. If garlic did not work well, it would have fallen out of the historical record some time ago. Instead, it has cemented itself in medical and human history, truly withstanding the test of time.

Since around the time of the Industrial Revolution the search for the chemical constituents of plant medicines began to appear. We got morphine from the opium poppy, ?uinine from chichona bark and aspirin from the willow. This is also the time work on garlic started. Scientists wanted to know why it worked and why garlic has its distinct smell when cut or crushed. They found contained in the garlic bulb a compound called allicin was made.

Allicin occurs by an enzymatic reaction when raw garlic is either crushed or somehow injured. The enzyme, alliinase, stored in a separate compartment in garlic, combines with a compound called alliin in raw garlic and produces allicin which has health enhancing properties. Allicin can break down into ajoene and the some 70 sulfur-containing garlic oils, most of which can help our health in a different way than allicin. These compounds make up a tiny fraction, only.1% to.36% of the total weight of a garlic bulb. Other compounds include water, carbohydrates, protein, fiber, vitamin A, B vitamins 1,2 and 3, vitamin C, zinc, calcium, manganese, germanium, selenium, copper, iron and adenosine (a nucleic acid).

A few points on these compounds. B1 is bound to the allicin, very rare in the plant kingdom. The combination called allithiamine is extremely easy to absorb and is used in Japan in nutritional supplements. Adenosine is a nucleic acid, a building block of DNA and RNA which contributes to garlic's beneficial effects on the blood; plus garlic contains more of this substance than any other plant food. Germanium and selenium minerals are both present in significant amounts which have been discussed in literature as being anticancer substances. The carbohydrates consist of at least 10 different sugars. One of these, scordinin, is regarded by the Japanese as a basic health enhancer. These eventually break down into a mixture of polysulfides which have no health or medical value. This means in a few weeks or months extracts will lose all their power unless protected in some way. Fresh garlic contains the most health benefits and boiling garlic completely removes all benefits.

Eating raw garlic is the best way to get garlic's benefits but the after effects on breath can cause the loss of friends, relatives and others close to you. Some people can get a temporary upset tummy from consuming raw garlic while others can get a rash from handling raw garlic. The freshest garlic is best for you but there's another thing to think about, garlic in stores is not fresh. Harvest time is usually between July and November. To get consistent potency and measured delivery of the beneficial materials, garlic should be consumed in a food supplement form.

Look for a pure, natural and pesticide free garlic product, preferably one that uses the cool-dry process. This will preserve as much of the active ingredients as possible. The label should state how much dried and fresh garlic is in each capsule or tablet. It should also tell you how many pills e?ual one clove of garlic; 1-2 cloves is usual for prevention of circulatory problems, 3 cloves is minimum for therapeutic effects such as antibacterial. It is also vital that the garlic you use has the distinct smell of garlic; the smell should be apparent when you break open a pill or capsule and/or put it into water.

Benefits Of Garlic

For generation, people are not only using garlic because of its medicinal value, but traditionally, people have rubbed their bodies with it, buried it besides their bodies in coffin, worn it around their necks, draped it on household walls and even prayed to it. This great bulb has a lot of benefits, because no other plant has been held out for so long as a cure for so many human ailments. That's why garlic has been considered as the "Wonder Drug".

Garlic has been used medicinally for many years for treating bites, tumors, ulcers, snakebite, wounds, headaches, heart diseases, cancer, pimples, measles and many more. It also prevents infections such as the common cold, cough because of its Anti-bacterial, Anti-fungal and Anti-viral property.

As this proverb is very common that

"An apple a day, keeps the doctor away".

In the same manner,

"A single bulb of garlic a day, keep diseases away".

In general, it exhibits antioxidant activity, which is good for your skin. It also contains flavonoids, which is good for heart and body.

"Allicin" in Garlic, which is a pungent oily liquid that gives crushed garlic cloves their characteristic smell, and has been shown to be the antibacterial agent due to its active sulphur.

Raw garlic is very smelly, so in order to reduce it smell, you can simply add it to your gravy, salad dressings, to soup, yummy pizza or just garnish it before serving or have it in your own style.

Tips:

Garlic is just magnificent and phenomenal. I am providing few of the basics known and reliable home remedies for some specific ailments, which you could try at your home .

If you have cold and flu, then take small amount of garlic every day until the infection disappears. Garlic tends to reduce the fre?uency of colds and flu without any side effects. A suggested dose would be two or three cloves of raw or cooked garlic a day.

We all face horrid acne, blemishes, blackheads during our teens. If you want to reduce it, or if you just want to glow up your skin, then take two cloves of raw garlic regularly with warm water early in the morning. It works as a blood cleanser and clean your system internally. Do not eat chocolates, spicy or oily food during this treatment and rinse your face five times a day with cold water. Drinks lots of water daily to flush off toxic waste from the blood and urinate whenever you feel that your bladder is full .Else, apply a cut clove gently on the affected area only if you have no sensitivity to it.

If you have High Cholesterol Level, use garlic in your food. This is the better way for heart patients to reduce their cholesterol level. Modern medical science suggests one reason that garlic might reduce cholesterol , i.e. "Garlic is a proven anti-oxidant". This property might help to prevent LDL (Low Density Lipo Protein) from being oxidized. In this way the cholesterol build-up that clogs the arteries could perhaps be reduced by garlic.

If you are very fat and want to loose weight, s?ueeze half lemon juice in one glass of luke warm water and drink it with two cloves of raw garlic regularly twice a day (morning and evening), for about three months. Avoid using starchy foods and fats. Do exercise regularly. You'll amazingly fell a great change in your body.

If you have Wrinkles, and you want to use anti ageing cream, it would be better to use 3 cloves of garlic regularly as it has a powerful antioxidant effect, which help to protect the body against damaging "Free Radicals". Remember, out skin is made up of collagen and it looses elasticity on yearly basis. Therefore, use garlic and do exercise regularly for the positive results.

If you have Earache, put two or three drops of warm garlic oil in the ears.

Take garlic to boosts the weight of babies in the womb. Thus, when they are born, they are heavier than they would have been if you hadn't taken garlic. Some babies are born too small, so garlic is a definite boon in these cases too.

Use two raw garlic daily to reduce the risk of cancer, due to its Anti-Carcinogenic properties. It helps prevent cancerous compounds from forming and developing into tumors. It also inhibits the growth of tumors.

If any insect bites you at the seaside, you just crush the garlic and apply it to the affected area to reduce pain and to remove poison.

How to take Garlic:

Crush two or three small cloves of raw garlic and eat it raw or boiled, before going to sleep. You can have it with a glass of milk or with water. Please do not take more than two or three raw cloves of garlic per day as it might makes your blood thinner and might cause serious ailments.

Contra-indications/precautions:

- Do not consume more than three to four raw cloves of garlic a day.
- Patients having heart and other problems should take medical advice before consuming it.
- It's best to avoid garlic before any surgery because it could probably disturb Anticoagulants.
- If you are on any medication, always check with your doctor first before taking raw garlic.
- Asthma patients should not use it as it worsens the symptoms of Asthma.
- If you have sensitive skin, I recommend not using physically on the affected area. Raw garlic can burn delicate skin! Do not use directly on skin if your skin is sensitive or susceptible to rashes or other skin reactions without consulting your doctor first. People who are or may be allergic to garlic or any of its sulfur compounds shouldn't try direct garlic application on skin too.

Side effect:

Although, garlic is a natural Anti-biotic but a very small number of people have been known to exhibit Hypersensitivity to garlic. Garlic allergy includes skin rash, temperature and headaches. Garlic intolerance could result in Heartburn or Flatulence.

Please note:

- It's important to remember that the effect of garlic on cold and flu comes from Allicin and this can be obtained from crushed, raw garlic and is destroyed by over cooking.

- Garlic cloves cooked whole have very little medicinal value.
- Garlic with strong smell has more Sulphur in it, which is good enough for medicinal purpose.

Facts about Garlic

- Garlic helps to boost up our Metabolism rate. Thus help us to reduce our weight easily.
- Garlic helps reduce Atherosclerotic buildup (Pla?ue) within the arterial system.
- Garlic lowers or helps to regulate Blood Sugar.
- Garlic helps to prevent blood clots from forming, thus reducing the possibility of Strokes.
- Garlic helps to prevent Cancer, especially of the digestive system, prevent certain tumors from growing larger and reduces the size of certain tumors.
- Garlic helps to remove heavy metals such as lead and mercury from the body.
- Raw garlic is a proven natural antibiotic and, while far less strong than modern antibiotics, can still kill some strains of bacteria that have become immune or resistant to modern antibiotics.
- Garlic dramatically reduces yeast infections in body parts.
- It helps to make our immune system stronger against cancer, ulcers, hemorrhoids etc

THREE

THE POWER OF GARLIC

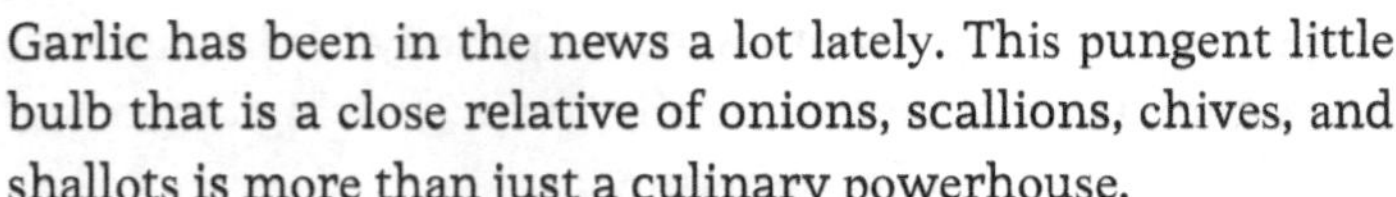

Garlic has been in the news a lot lately. This pungent little bulb that is a close relative of onions, scallions, chives, and shallots is more than just a culinary powerhouse.

The healing power of garlic has a long historical tradition. Garlic has been cultivated for at least 5,000 years. The early Egyptians ate it and used it as a medicine. Romans used garlic to treat asthma, suppress coughs, and expel intestinal parasites. Ancient Chinese physicians utilized garlic to reduce fevers and fight against intestinal parasites and dysentery.

Over the centuries, herbalists in many countries have used garlic as an antibacterial, antifungal, antioxidant, anti-inflammatory, and immune-stimulant.

In the mid-nineteenth century, scientist Louis Pasteur noted the antibiotic properties of garlic when he put a small piece of the herb in a petri dish of bacteria, which it quickly killed. Scientific evidence supporting the role of garlic as a potent botanical medicine has accumulated since that time.

Fresh garlic, used as food and medicine, has a history that dates back to at least 5000 years. It is bursting with antioxidants known to prevent heart disease, cancer and anti-ageing. It is cheap, safe and easily available throughout the whole year. For the busy cooks, garlic powder, garlic salad seasonings and spicy garlic sauce can easily be bought online.

Garlic has antibiotic and anti-inflammatory properties. It improves digestion and eliminates worm. Garlic with its antiviral properties, can be used to treat tonsillitis Prepare crushed or minced garlic at least ten minutes before using it to preserve its disease fighting properties. Using garlic as a whole bulb during cooking loses some of these diseases fighting properties. Having difficulty eating raw garlic? Garlic can be easily included into your everyday meals.

Some common uses for garlic are as follows:

1. Mix juice from crushed garlic with honey to prevent stomach ulcers and coughs.
2. Chewing pips of garlic helps to prevent tapeworm infection.
3. Eating garlic raw is said to help in the body's immunity against diseases.

Modern Research on Garlic

During the past twenty-five years, medical research has documented that garlic consumption reduces cholesterol and triglycerides in the blood while increasing lipoproteins (good cholesterol).

Garlic tends to lower high blood pressure. Some studies even suggest that garlic may help prevent cancer and diabetes. However, a recent major study, based on a comprehensive review of the medical literature, analyzed the potential medical value of garlic and concluded that the advocates for this strong smelling herb may have overstated the case for its effectiveness. The report by the Agency for Healthcare Research and Quality calls for additional research to examine the short-term versus long-term benefits of regular garlic consumption.

FOUR

ANTI-AGING SUPERFOOD

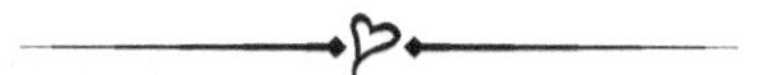

Is garlic good as anti-ageing? Absolutely! A diet that contains plenty of garlic, especially raw garlic, can go a long way towards preventing pre-mature wrinkles and fine lines on aging skin. The wrinkle fighting properties associated with garlic use are primarily attributed to allicin, a natural compound that is produced when raw garlic is crushed or chopped. Allicin has been touted as one of the world's most powerful antioxidants.

Antioxidants such as allicin inhibit free radical activity, which in turn helps fight wrinkles and fine lines provoked by an overdose of skin-damaging UV radiation. When your skin is exposed to the sun's UV rays, your body responds by forming enzymes called metalloproteinases. Some of these enzymes break down connective tissue — which can eventually lead to wrinkles and fine lines — and free radicals are known to boost production of harmful metalloproteinases.

In addition to delivering allicin, raw garlic is good for fighting wrinkles because it provides plenty of antioxidant minerals such as zinc and selenium. Furthermore, raw garlic is loaded with vitamin C, and ounce for ounce, it contains more than twice as much vitamin C as fresh tomatoes. While vitamin C is best known for its ability to scavenge wrinkle causing free radicals, it can also prevent pre-mature wrinkling of the skin by supporting healthy collagen production. As an added beauty benefit, vitamin C can help with pigmentation problems and inflammatory skin conditions.

Here are a few ways in which you can use garlic to get clean and glowing skin

1. Acne, Pimples And Spot Treatment

As I already mentioned, allicin has antifungal properties which can be used to get rid of those stubborn acne that have been giving you sleepless nights.

a. Just cut a freshly piece of raw garlic and apply a little pressure on it to release some juice and then rub this garlic pod onto the affected area. Leave it for 5 minutes and was off with cold water. You'll see a reduction in redness and swelling within the day. Also, this helps in prevention of acne leaving behind marks on your skin.

b. Another simple techni?ue to get rid of acne using garlic is mixing juice from 2-3 pods of garlic with an equal ?uantity of white vinegar and applying it to the affected area. The white vinegar helps in maintaining the skin's pH levels while garlic fights infection.

c. c. For those who can't bear the sting that raw garlic causes when used alone, peel a few garlic pods and crush them. Add half tsp. honey and 2 tbsp. yogurt. Apply this mask all over the face and wash within 20 minutes. Instead of using raw garlic you can also use garlic oil or garlic powder. Both these variants are easily available in the market. Never use more than 2-3 drops of garlic oil and half teaspoon of garlic powder.

d. To get rid of acne scaring and blemishes, make a paste by taking 4-5 pieces of peeled raw garlic and whacking each one with a mallet so that it breaks open. Do not mince this completely. Boil 250 ml of water and as soon as it comes to a boil, add the garlic. Boil the garlic for 30-35 minutes and make sure that the garlic is always submerged in water. When the garlic has finished boiling, let it cool till it is lukewarm. Now use your mallet or a rolling pin to make a garlic paste and apply this paste liberally on your entire face. The boiling ensures that the garlic is not too strong for the skin.

2. Blackhead And Whitehead Removal

One of the most common skin problems is blackheads. Their occurrence is particularly very high when you have oily skin.

a. Take 2-3 cloves garlic and crush them. Add 1 tbsp. of oatmeal, 1-2 drops of tea tree oil and half tsp. lemon juice. Mix these ingredients with honey to form a thick paste. Spread a thin layer of this paste onto clean skin. After letting it sit for 2-3 minutes, gently exfoliate your face followed by a rinse with warm water. Use this mask thrice in a week to see a visible reduction in blackheads.

3. Anti-ageing And Pore Minimization

Garlic beauty benefits also include the aid for anti aging. The strong anti-oxidants present in garlic help in reducing the free radical build up in the skin thus keeping it firm and youthful. It also contains sulphur, which helps the body to produce collagen which inturn helps in fighting wrinkles. Garlic also contains a large number of skin-protective polyphenols. Just crush some garlic pods and add the juice into your regular face masks for added goodness and preventing premature aging.

a. Enlarged pores are a common problem in ageing skin. To minimize pores make a paste by mashing together half a tomato and 3-4 pods of garlic. Spread a thin layer of the paste onto your face. After 20 minutes, wash your face with lukewarm water and seal your pores with a final splash of cold water. Tomato and garlic both have antiseptic ?ualities that help in unclogging the skin, minimizes pores and tightens the skin.

b. Consuming pill-size pieces of garlic every day also works great to protect the skin from damages caused by free radicals, oxidation, and environmental stressors that eventually results in wrinkles.

4. Stretch Mark Removal

There are not many things that you can do to prevent stretch marks from appearing but garlic can definitely help you in getting rid of them. Stretch marks are known to reduce and vanish if you use garlic.

a. a. Hot oil massage is one of the most commonly suggested home remedy for this problem. To make more effective, add juice from crushed garlic pods in the hot oil that you use. Use this oil regularly on your stretch marks and you will notice the difference in a few weeks. Instead of using garlic juice, you can also use garlic oil. Do take care not to add more than half tsp. of garlic oil.

b.   Also increase consumption of garlic in your diet as the allicin and sulphur in garlic are known to increase the elasticity of the skin which prevents the stretch marks from occurring

5. Garlic Benefits For Hair

Garlic is excellent for hair growth. It helps in decreasing hair fall, boosts regeneration of new hair follicles, removes harmful toxins from the scalp, enhances hair texture, and reinforces the hair roots.

The allicin in garlic helps in increasing blood circulation in the scalp which in turn reduces hair fall and helps in stimulating hair growth. Garlic also has anti-bacterial and anti-fungal properties that help in treating dandruff and itchy scalp. The sulphur present in garlic reduces the severity of dandruff and prevents it from coming back.

a.   The simplest way to use garlic for hair is to add a clove of garlic in either your shampoo or conditioner. But make sure that you don't use the garlic shampoo or conditioner more than twice a month as excessive use of garlic can cause dryness of scalp and hair. To get rid of the overpowering smell and slight tingling sensation that garlic causes, add honey along with garlic when you add it to your conditioner. Honey will also work as a natural conditioner for your hair.

b.   To reduce hair fall, soak a handful of garlic cloves in olive oil for a week. After a week, use this oil to massage your scalp and leave it overnight and wash your hair as usual.

Use this oil once a week and you will notice a reduction
in hair fall.

c. To avoid grey hair, heat some coconut oil and add a few
dry black pepper seeds and 3 cloves of garlic. When it cools
apply this oil to your hair. Use this hair oil continuously
for a few days to note the difference.

6. Garlic Benefits For Nails

The benefits of garlic are not only restricted to skin and
hair. Garlic can also help you in getting rid of dull and brittle
nails. As it has anti-bacterial properties, it also helps in
preventing any kind of cuticle infection.

a. To get rid of yellowness of nails, do the following. Whack
garlic clove using a mallet to release the juice and rub this
clove all over your fingernails. Repeat this twice a week
and you will have long and strong nails in no time.

b. You can also add a few drops of garlic oil or garlic juice in
your regular cuticle cream or lotion to reap the benefits
garlic has to offer whenever you apply these to your nails.

7. Supports Body Metabolism

Another huge benefit of garlic is that the sulphur in garlic
works with B complex vitamins and support body
metabolism, which in turn helps in keeping the healthy
which shows on your skin and hair and also helps with
weight loss. Take juice of half a lemon and mix it with
lukewarm water and consume it with two cloves of garlic
twice a day for 2-3 months to see results.

FIVE

CAUTIONS

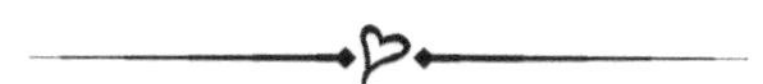

Garlic isn't recommended in all situations. Consider safety tips and cautions before use.

- Do not give garlic supplements to children. Consult physician, first.
- Consult your health care provider before use, especially, if you have plant allergies.
- Do not take garlic supplements when pregnant or breast-feeding, since its effects on unborn or nursing infants are unknown.
- Raw garlic can have side effects: bad breath, burning sensation in mouth or stomach, heartburn, gas, nausea, vomiting, body odor and diarrhea.
- Can increase or prolong the risk of bleeding. It can affect blood clotting and blood sugar levels. Consult your health care provider before taking garlic, if you have a bleeding or blood clotting disorder or diabetes. Consult your health care provider if on blood thinning or other medications.

SIX

CONCLUSION

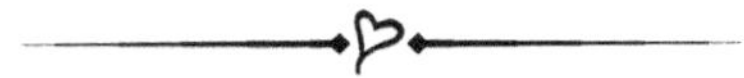

For generation, people are not only using garlic because of its medicinal value, but traditionally, people have rubbed their bodies with it, buried it besides their bodies in coffin, worn it around their necks, draped it on household walls and even prayed to it. This great bulb has a lot of benefits, because no other plant has been held out for so long as a cure for so many human ailments. That's why garlic has been considered as the "Super food".

Disclaimer

Introduction

By using this book, you accept this disclaimer in full.

No advice

The book contains information. The information is not advice and should not be treated as such.

No representations or warranties

To the maximum extent permitted by applicable law and subject to section below, we exclude all representations, warranties, undertakings and guarantees relating to the book.

Without prejudice to the generality of the foregoing paragraph, we do not represent, warrant, undertake or guarantee:

- that the information in the book is correct, accurate, complete or non-misleading.

- that the use of the guidance in the book will lead to any particular outcome or result.

Limitations and exclusions of liability

The limitations and exclusions of liability set out in this section and elsewhere in this disclaimer: are subject to section 6 below; and govern all liabilities arising under the disclaimer or in relation to the book, including liabilities arising in contract, in tort (including negligence) and for breach of statutory duty.

We will not be liable to you in respect of any losses arising out of any event or events beyond our reasonable control.

We will not be liable to you in respect of any business losses, including without limitation loss of or damage to profits, income, revenue, use, production, anticipated savings, business, contracts, commercial opportunities or goodwill.

We will not be liable to you in respect of any loss or corruption of any data, database or software.

We will not be liable to you in respect of any special, indirect or consequential loss or damage.

Exceptions

Nothing in this disclaimer shall: limit or exclude our liability for death or personal injury resulting from negligence; limit or exclude our liability for fraud or fraudulent misrepresentation; limit any of our liabilities in any way that is not permitted under applicable law; or exclude any of our liabilities that may not be excluded under applicable law.

Severability

If a section of this disclaimer is determined by any court or other competent authority to be unlawful and/ or unenforceable, the other sections of this disclaimer continue in effect.

If any unlawful and/or unenforceable section would be lawful or enforceable if part of it were deleted, that part will be deemed to be deleted, and the rest of the section will continue in effect.

Law and jurisdiction

This disclaimer will be governed by and construed in accordance with Swiss law, and any disputes relating to this disclaimer will be subject to the exclusive jurisdiction of the courts of Switzerland.